101 Tips On Losing
10 Pounds

Look Slim And Sexy After Losing 10 Pounds Now!

By: Samantha Michaels

TABLE OF CONTENTS

PUBLISHERS NOTES

DEDICATION

This book is dedicated to individuals who desire to lose weight.

Tips 1 to 20

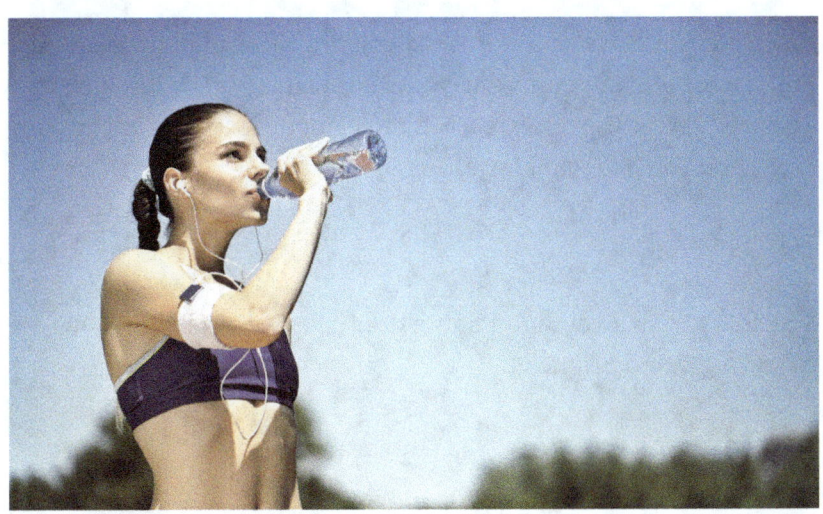

Tip # 1

Drink plenty of water. Water is not just way to flush out toxins. If you have more water in your body you will generally feel healthier and fitter. It also helps you feel full, so you don't have the urge to eat so much. And water has no calories at all.

Tip # 2

Start your day with a glass of water. It's a wonderful way to start you day. A glass of water lubricates your insides. You can still have your morning cup of tea, but have it after a glass of water.

Tip # 3

Drink a glass of water before you eat each meal. Water takes up space in your stomach, so you feel fuller without eating as much.

Tip # 4

Have another glass of water while you are having your meal. Again this is another way of making yourself full. Instead of drinking it all at once, take a sip after each bite of food. It will help the food settle and you'll feel full faster.

Tip # 5

Stay away from sweetened bottle drinks, especially sodas. They are full of sugar and calories.

Tip # 6

Include foods that contain more water, like tomatoes and watermelons. They contain 90 - 95 % water, so feast on them as much as you like. They fill you up without adding pounds.

Tip # 7

Eat fresh fruit instead of drinking fruit juice. Juice is often sweetened with sugar, but fresh fruit has natural sugars. When you eat fruit, you are taking in a lot of fiber, which the body needs, and fruit is an excellent source of vitamins.

Tip # 8

If you have a craving for fruit juice, try making your own. There are lots of juicing machines on the market.

Tip # 9

Choose fresh fruit instead of processed fruit. Processed and canned fruit does not have as much fiber as fresh fruit and processed and canned fruit is nearly always sweetened with sugar.

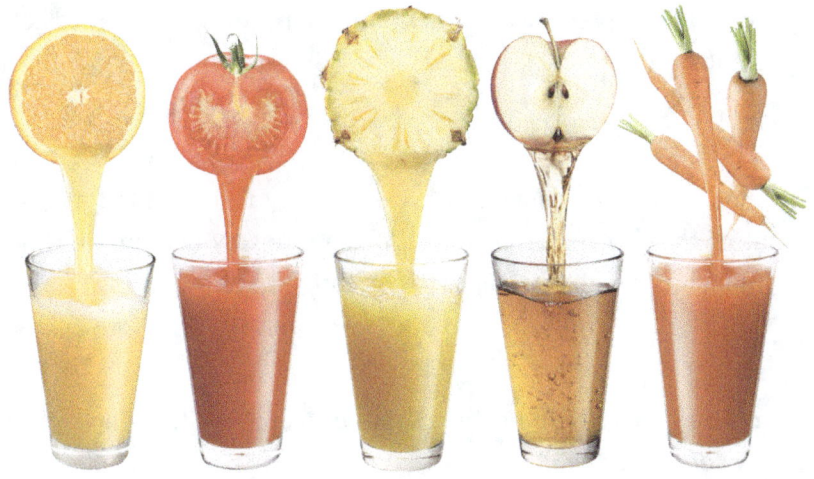

Tip # 10

Increase your fiber intake. Your body needs a lot of fiber, so try to include it in your diet. Eat as many fruits and vegetables as you can.

Tip # 11

Eat lots of vegetables. Leafy green vegetables are the best. Include a salad in your meal plan every day.

Tip # 12

Eat intelligently. Choose your foods wisely. Instead of grabbing chips or candy bars, grab a fruit or vegetable.

Tip # 13

Watch what you eat. Sometimes the garnishes can be richer than the food itself. Accompaniments can be very rich too.

Tip # 14

Control your sweet tooth. Sweets generally mean calories. You don't have to cut sweets out of your diet completely, but eat them in moderation. Every sweet you put in your mouth adds fat cells to your body.

Tip # 15

Develop a meal schedule and stick to it. Try to have food at fixed times of the day. You can stretch these times by half an hour, but anything more is going to affect your eating pattern.

Tip # 16

Eat only when you are hungry. Some of us have a tendency to eat whenever we see food.

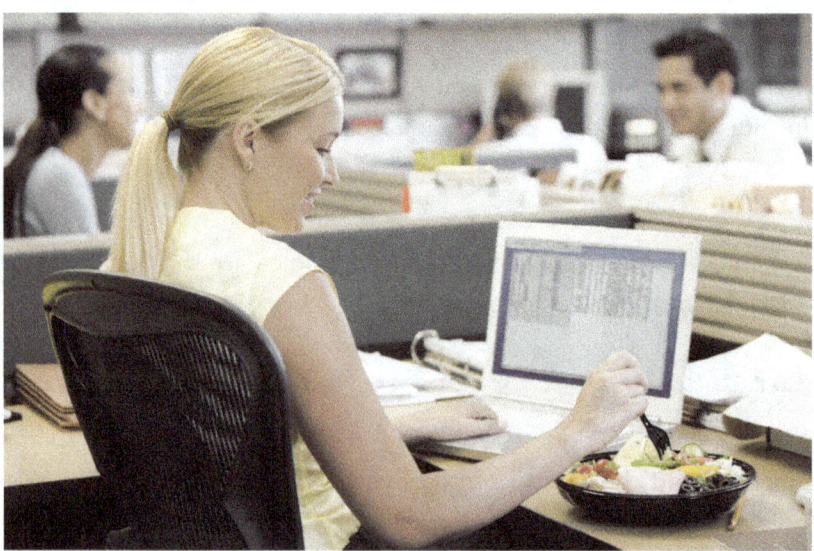

Tip # 17

Quit snacking between meals. The main problem with most snacks and junk food is, they are usually less filling and contain a lot of fat and calories.

Tip # 18

Snack on vegetables if you have to snack.

Tip # 19

Go easy on tea and coffee. Tea and coffee are harmless by themselves, but when you add cream and sugar they become fattening. Having a cup of tea or coffee with cream and sugar is as bad as having a piece of chocolate cake.

Tip # 20

Drink black tea/coffee. Black tea or coffee can actually be good for you. But personally I would like to recommend tea rather than coffee. The caffeine in the coffee is not really good for you because it is an alkaloid and can affect other functions of your body like the metabolism.

TIPS 21 TO 40

Tip # 21

Count the calories as you eat. Check the label of any packaged product for the number of calories and the serving size. For unpackaged food, buy a calorie counting book.

Tip # 22

If you consume more calories than you should one day, add a bit of extra physical activity to your routine for the following day.

Tip # 23

Stay away from fried foods. The oil used for frying penetrates into the food and adds unwanted calories.

Tip # 24

Do not skip meals. The worst thing you can do while watching your weight is skip a meal. It has just the opposite effect of what you want. You need to have at least three regular meals every day.

Tip # 25

Fresh vegetables are better than cooked or canned vegetables. Try to eat your vegetables raw. When you cook them, you are removing nearly half the vitamins.

Tip # 26

One egg a day. It's best if you reduce your egg intake to three a week. If you're in the habit of eating eggs every day, limit your eggs to one a day maximum.

Tip # 27

Make chocolates a luxury and not a routine.

Tip # 28

Choose a variety of foods from all food groups every day. In addition to helping you lose weight, it also helps your body fight deficiency diseases. Change the foods you eat each day so you do not get bored of your diet.

Tip # 29

Very limited or no alcoholic beverages.

Tip # 30

Try to have breakfast within one hour of waking up, so your body can charge itself with the energy it needs for the day. Breakfast is the most important meal of the day, but it does not mean that it should be the most filling meal of the day.

Tip # 31

50% - 55% of your diet should be carbohydrates. It is a myth that you should try and avoid carbohydrates when you are on a diet. Carbohydrates are an instant source of energy.

Tip # 32

25% - 30% of your diet should be proteins. Protein is an active part of keeping your body healthy.

Tip # 33

Fats should only be 15% - 20 % of your diet

Tip # 34

Try and adopt a vegetarian style diet. A vegetarian diet is healthy, but research has shown it often is missing vital minerals that come from eating meat. If you try a vegetarian diet, allow yourself to eat meat on the weekends.

Tip # 35

Choose white meat rather than red. White meat, which includes fish and fowl, is healthier than red meat.

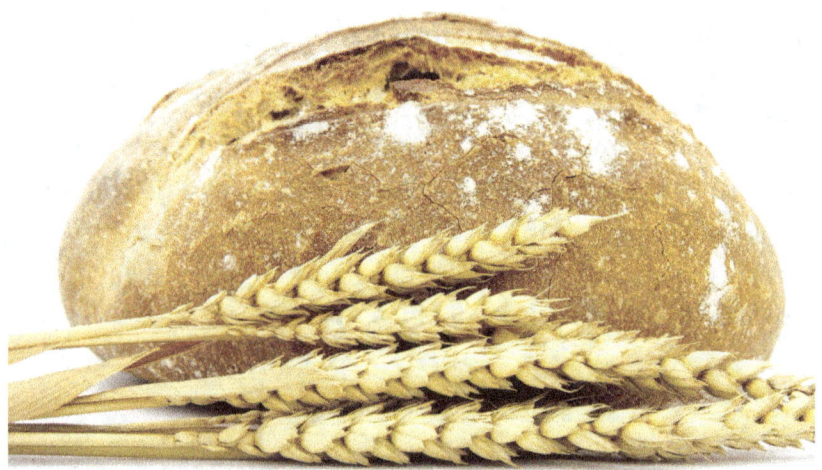

Tip # 36

High Fiber multigrain breads are better than white breads. Multigrain breads allow you to increase your fiber and protein intake.

Tip # 37

Reduce your intake of pork. Pork is not something that can help you to lose weight. So the lesser pork you eat the better chances you have of losing weight. And remember that pork includes the pork products as well, things like bacon, ham and sausages.

Tip # 38

Limit your sugar intake. Use sugar substitutes to sweeten your food. They are just as sweetening, but not fattening.

Tip # 39

Graze 5 to 6 times a day. Instead of sticking to just three meals a day, try grazing. Grazing means having 5 or 6 smaller meals instead of three large meals. It is an excellent way of having smaller quantities of food.

Tip # 40

Eat cheat food occasionally, but only for flavor. There are many foods you need to avoid in your diet, but you may have an undying craving for them. Do not avoid them altogether. Indulge in them once in a while, but only in moderation. Don't use them to fill up, but simply to fill a craving. Enjoy the flavor.

TIPS 41 TO 60

Tip # 41

Watch your fat intake. Each fat gram contains 9 calories. By knowing the total calories and the quantity of fat in your food, you can estimate the percentage of fat. Fat content should not exceed 30%.

Tip # 42

Go easy on salt. Too much salt is one of the causes of obesity.

Tip # 43

Change from butter to cholesterol free butter. It tastes the same, but is much healthier for you.

Tip # 44

Instead of frying food, try baking it. Baking is a healthier method of preparing food because it doesn't require excessive amounts of fat or oil.

Tip # 45

Use a non-stick frying pan for your cooking so you do not have to add oil.

Tip # 46

Steam your vegetables instead of cooking them. The best option is eating your vegetables fresh, however, if you do not like eating fresh vegetables, try steaming them without adding any additional salt or seasoning. This is the healthiest way to eat cabbages, cauliflowers and a host of other vegetables.

Tip # 47

Carry parsley with you. Parsley is an excellent thing to munch on between meals. It's vitamin rich and keeps your breath fresh.

Tip # 48

Choose low fat or no fat substitutes. Although fat gives us nutrients, it also packs on the calories. It's much better to get your nutrients from proteins and carbohydrates. It's healthier for your heart too.

Tip # 49

Avoid crash diets. They are bad for your health and you will gain your weight back as soon as you stop them. Crash diets are not a solution to weight loss. You might lose a few pounds quickly, but the moment you give up on the crash diet, all your weight comes back.

Tip # 50

Develop a habit of chewing all your food including liquid food and soft foods like sweets, and ice cream, at least 8 to 12 times. This is essential to add saliva to the food, as it starts the digestion process.

Tip # 51

Dry wine is better than sweet wine. Sweet wines naturally contain a lot of sugar, but in dry wines, most of the sugar has been fermented away.

Tip # 52

When you decide it's time to start working out, start slowly and don't get discouraged if you don't achieve your fitness goals after the first week. If you try to push your body too much in the first few weeks, you are likely to end up with injuries.

Tip # 53

Check your weight before you start a training routine and keep checking for changes, but do not expect a radical drop immediately. It might be a couple weeks before you notice some change. However it is crucial that you continue to monitor your weight. As you're losing fat weight, you're gaining muscle mass, so your overall weight may not change as dramatically as you would like it to. Your size, however, will decrease, so measure your body regularly too.

Tip # 54

When you notice a change, reward yourself but not with food. Go to a movie or buy yourself something like a new dress or accessories. This can help keep you motivated.

Tip # 55

Take a day off from exercise every week. Your body needs a day or two each week to relax and rejuvenate itself.

Tip # 56

Exercise outdoors as much as possible. It gives your body a chance to get fresh air and sunshine. It also keeps you perked up and it's a break from being inside all day.

Tip # 57

Exercise at home. You don't need to join a gym to exercise. You don't even need to buy exercise equipment. Visit the library or look online for exercises you can do without equipment. If you do want to get some equipment, a Wii Fit is a great investment and it makes exercising a lot of fun.

Tip # 58

Exercise with a friend. Ideally, it should be somebody committed to exercising like you or your interest might fade.

Tip # 59

Stop when your body has had enough. There is no need to push it. When you have worked out for a considerable time, your body will start giving you signals.

Listen to your body, especially in the initial stages. Take one step at a time. Stop when you are out of breath or when a certain part of your body tells you that it has had enough.

Tip # 60

Increase your exercise time gradually. Dramatic jumps in exercise time can leave your body exhausted and more prone to injury. Instead of increasing your workout routine by 30 minutes, increase it by 10 minutes a week for 3 weeks.

TIPS 61 TO 80

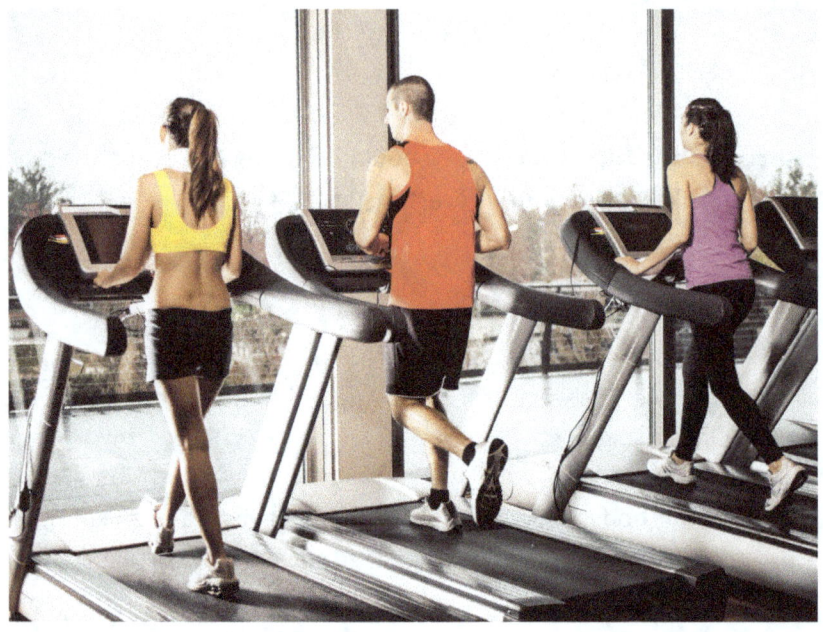

Tip # 61

Select an exercise pattern to suit your lifestyle. All of us have different lifestyles and professions so follow an exercise routine that is suitable for you.

Tip # 62

Don't stand, walk. If you can walk about then do so. Do not stand in a fixed position. Pacing about is a good thing to do. If you are thinking deeply about something, try pacing, it will aid in your thinking too.

Tip # 63

Don't sit, stand. If you can stand, then do not sit. The golden rule is to choose a position that is less comfortable.

Tip # 64

Don't lie down, sit. The rule that we mentioned above rings true here as well.

Tip # 65

Replace the comfortable couch and chairs in front of the TV. If you have less comfortable furniture in front of the TV, you are less likely to sit in front of it.

Tip # 66

If you have a sitting job, stand up and stretch every half hour. Most jobs today are sitting jobs that are sedentary. By stretching every half hour you help your body stay awake and your metabolism running, which helps burn fat.

Tip # 67

While making telephone calls try walking around.

Tip # 68

Use the stairs instead of the elevator whenever you can. If you have to travel to the 40th floor, take the elevator part way and walk the rest of the way.

Tip # 69

Smoking is bad for weight loss. Smoking may not contribute to weight loss but smoking leads to other conditions like erratic eating habits and excessive dependence on things like coffee.

Tip # 70

If you hate running, remember, you do not have to run a marathon to stay fit. 10 minutes of cardio each day is good enough for most people.

Tip # 71

If you can't run, try walking. 15 minutes of brisk walking a day is enough to keep most people fit.

Tip # 72

Any distance is walkable if you have the time, so consider walking to places that you would normally drive, such as work or the market if they're not too far away. It may take you longer, but the health benefits will last you a lifetime.

Tip # 73

It sounds strange, but some people have reported that they lost more weight when they drank black coffee before a workout. While there's no hard data to support this, nutritionists speculate that the caffeine in coffee makes the body rely more on fat for fuel during the work out. It's worth trying.

Tip # 74

Avoid drinking coffee in excess, as it tends to desensitize your body to the fat burning effects of caffeine.

Tip # 75

Stop using remote controls. Get up from the couch and change the TV channel manually.

Tip # 76

Often when we come home tired from work, we tend to get others to do simple chores for us. These things are no big deal. They are things that we can do for ourselves, but we don't.

Tip # 77

Walk up and down escalators as if they were normal stairs.

Tip # 78

During TV commercial breaks, get up and walk around. Reach over and touch your toes or do any simple exercise that will get the blood flowing.

Tip # 79

Wriggle your toes and your fingers whenever you can. This is a stress reliever and it gives you a chance to work your hand and leg joints.

Tip # 80

Turn on music and dance like wild. Let your hair down once in a while. Think back to the days of your wild child hood. Close the door of your room, turn on your sound system to the highest volume possible and do the wackiest dance you can think of. Jump on your bed and jump off it again. Roll all over the floor. Have fun.

TIPS 81 TO 101

Tip # 81

Carry a soft flying disc or Frisbee with you. Toss it around and get up and go get it. This is also an excellent way to beat stress. It makes you feel good to throw something. Although it's not the throwing part that you are interested in, it is the fetching part. Each time you get up to fetch, you are giving yourself a chance to stretch your muscles and joints and get your metabolism working harder to burn more fat.

Tip # 82

Park at least a block away from your destination and walk the rest of the way. You might not have time to fit long walks into your busy schedule, so this is a way to ensure you get to walk for a little bit every day. If you take the bus or the subway, get off at an earlier station and walk the rest of the way.

Tip # 83

When nobody is watching try doing pelvic gyrations. Your mid-section gets the least bit of exercise so excess weight tends to settle there.

Stomach crunches might be too strenuous an exercise to start off with, but gyrations are relatively mild. Pelvic gyrations make you thrust your midsection towards all directions and this is the best way of tightening every muscle in that area.

Tip # 84

Tuck in your tummy whenever you walk. Get that proper gait and exercise your muscles at the same time.

Tip # 85

Try breathing exercises. Breathing exercises can lead to weight loss. If you are doing the breathing exercises properly, you will find that you can exert a lot of pressure on the muscles around the mid-section.

You can feel a tightening of these muscles each time you breathe in or breathe out. So breathe properly, it is good for you.

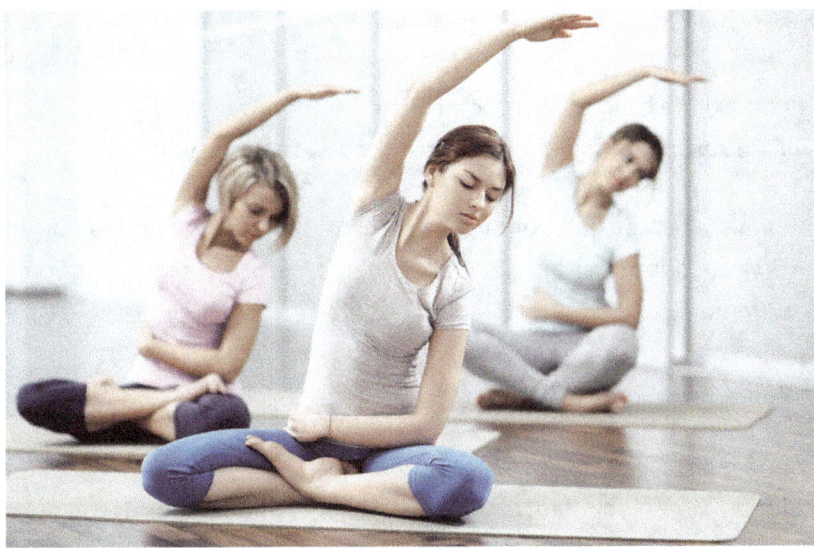

Tip # 86

Try yoga. Yoga is one of the best ways of losing weight. One of the benefits of yoga is, you learn to control virtually every muscle and joint of your body so the issue of weight gain will cease to exist.

Tip # 87

Try massaging your partner. This is a fun way to lose weight. It is something that can give your partner a lot of pleasure and at the same time can help you exercise.

Tip # 88

Punch the air 50 times. It helps your cardiovascular system and jump starts your metabolism.

Tip # 89

Instead of walking up and down the stairs one at a time, take them two at a time.

Tip # 90

If you have a dog, take it for a run and let the dog lead you on. You will be surprised how much exercise a dog can give you.

Animals are sensible enough to know that they need a lot of exercise, so let your animal walk you and before you know it you'll be running.

Tip # 91

Join a dance class. Dancing is a wonderful way to burn off extra calories. When you dance, you are burning a lot of calories.

Tip # 92

Lean against a wall with your hands flat against the wall and your face very close to the wall. Use your hands to push your body away from the wall. It resembles a standing push up and is easier than lying on the floor.

Tip # 93

If there is a pool nearby, go for a swim as often as you can. Swimming is one of the best exercises to move your whole body.

Tip # 94

Play table tennis or basketball. Games are a fun way to lose weight. It is much more exciting to play a game than just work out by yourself. The best thing about games is, they are addictive. It is something you can look forward to and there is no stress involved in the program. In fact the more you play the less you will consider this to be a part of your weight loss program. As you burn away those calories, you will also be able to expand your social circle.

Tip # 95

Any work out should start with a 5 to 10 minute warm up and should end with a 5 to 10 minute cool down session. Your body needs to reach a certain level of readiness before it can actually start responding to exercise.

Tip # 96

Do not carry your mobile phone, but leave it someplace where you can hear it ringing. When it rings, you have to get up to answer it.

Tip # 97

While traveling in an elevator, raise up on your toes and then back onto your feet again. Do this several times. Also try flexing your buttock muscles.

In fact there are many muscles in our body that we can twitch and flex without inviting the attention of others. Even if others do notice you, its no big deal.

Tip # 98

Undress and stare at yourself in front of your mirror. If what you see displeases you, then you have more reason to work out.

Turn to your side and get a very good view of your side profile. This is an excellent way of checking whether you have a tummy that is starting to bulge or has bulged already.

Tip # 99

If you have a banister rail or a balustrade that will support you, sit on it and pump your legs as if you are riding a bicycle, taking care not to fall off. This might sound like a crazy idea, but it's fun. And fun will keep you active.

Tip # 100

Do not slouch in your chair. Maintain an erect posture with your tummy tucked in. Slouching is a very bad habit. Not only is it bad for your back, but it also gives you a very flabby figure.

Tip # 101

Breathe in as strongly as you can and tuck in your tummy as much as you can. Hold it for a few seconds and slowly release your breath, taking care not to let out your tummy. Try to keep breathing like this at least fifty or sixty times a day.

After the first day, you should feel the muscles of your stomach tightening each time you do this. Practice this for 20 days. At the end of the twentieth day, you will have lost at least an inch.

BONUS

Below I have included a table of the various exercises and the number of calories that can be burnt with each exercise. Choose what you can do best and choose something that you will enjoy doing in the long run.

The choice of exercise is completely up to you, but do whatever you wish for at least twenty minutes. It is only after you do the exercise for twenty minutes that the actual calorie burning sets in.

Aerobics	200-250 Calories
Bicycling, Stationary	250-300 Calories
Bicycling, Actual	300-400 Calories
Running, 5-6 mph	300-350 Calories
Stair Climber	200-250 Calories
Swimming Laps	350 Calories
Walking Briskly	150-180 Calories

How Much Do You Know?

From the information you just read, how much do you remember?

1) Which of the following is suitable for a between meal snack?

   A. Cheese
   B. Carrots
   C. Yogurt
   D. Coffee
   E. Candy

2) How many glasses of water should a person have in a day?

   A. 5-6
   B. 10-20
   C. 10- 12
   D. 4-5
   E. 15-20

3) Which of the following is bad as far as weight control is concerned?

   A. Snacking
   B. Smoking
   C. Coffee
   D. Crash diets
   E. All the above

4) How many hours sleep does an adult need?

A. 7-8
B. 6-7
C. 8-9
D. 5-6
E. 9-10

5) Which is better for a person on a diet?

A. Fresh Fruit
B. Canned Fruit
C. Fruit Juice
D. Processed Fruit
E. Cooked Fruit

6) Which of the following should you always include in your diet?

A. Nuts
B. Dried Fruits
C. Fruit Juice
D. Salads
E. Tea

7) Which is better for your health?

A. Coffee
B. Tea

8) The most important meal of the day is

A. Supper
B. Snacks
C. Breakfast
D. Lunch
E. Tea

9) Which of the following can you afford to cut out from your diet?

A. Fats
B. Carbohydrates
C. Vegetables
D. Proteins
E. Vitamins

10) Which meat is better for you?

A. White Meat
B. Red Meat
C. Raw Meat

Answers:

1. B
2. C
3. E
4. A
5. A
6. D
7. B
8. C
9. A
10. A

Samantha Michaels

Muscle Power

Use your brain to answer the test on the best ways to work out.

1.) Which is the best exercise?

    A. Horse Riding
    B. Walking
    C. Swimming
    D. Running
    E. Bowling

2.) Before you work out, you need to

    A. Drink Water
    B. Warm Up
    C. Consult A Trainer
    D. Make Up Your Mind
    E. Cool Off

3.) You can afford to take a day off from your work out every week

    A. True
    B. False

4.) Yoga does not help to reduce weight

    A. True
    B. False

5.) Breathing exercises strengthen the shoulder muscles

    A. True
    B. False

Answers:

1. C
2. B
3. A
4. A
5. B

Conclusion

Eating a balanced diet and increasing your physical activity will help you reduce your weight. Drink extra water each day and ensure you are eating fruit and vegetables and you'll begin to see results very quickly.

ABOUT THE AUTHOR

Samantha Michaels has spent years helping people overcome health challenges, lose weight and reach ideal health goals while enjoying good and healthy food. She is an author of numerous health books and provide amazing yet very healthy recipes everyone can enjoy.

She loves food and spends most of her time helping people address diet challenges by teaching them to cook the right meals. Her diet programs have helped a lot of people lose weight in a smart, practical way and she lives what she preaches that you do not have to get hungry while on a diet.

www.ingramcontent.com/pod-product-compliance
Lightning Source LLC
Chambersburg PA
CBHW061942280526
45787CB00004B/1690